The Best Cri◖

2021-2022

A detailed and updated step-by-step guide to learning how to use every Cricut Design Space tool and function, with illustrations.

Table of Contents

INTRODUCTION

Is it accurate to say that you are attempting to get the hang of everything about Cricut Design Space and you don't realize where to begin?

Learning another pastime or aptitude can be scary from the start. I get it, now and then we don't realize where to begin because there's such a great amount of data out there and it's simply overpowering.

For me, the ideal approach to learn and ace Cricut Design Space is from the earliest starting point!

When you have a reasonable idea of what each symbol and board is for, then you can genuinely dive in and begin investigating further and further.

Once in a while, we rush to bounce from undertaking to extend – Hey That's alright as well! BTDT – But I feel that knowing your work zone will assist you with taking your imagination in an unheard of level.

My Cricut machine is experiencing difficulty understanding cartridges

If you are getting cartridge mistake messages when utilizing your Cricut machine remain solitary, or if the machine isn't perusing the cartridges by any stretch of the imagination, if it's not too much trouble select your machine from the connections underneath and pursue the suggested investigating steps.

Cricut Personal, Cricut Create, Cricut Cake, Cricut Cake Mini, Cricut Expression

Cricut Expression 2

Cricut Imagine

Cricut Personal, Cricut Create, Cricut Cake, Cricut Cake Mini, Cricut Expression

Offer the Cricut a reprieve; turn the Cricut off and enable it to rest for around 10 minutes every hour.

Evacuate the cartridge and set it back in reverse. It is conceivable that the stickers were inappropriately put on the cartridge.

Have a go at utilizing a different cartridge. If the Cricut never again demonstrates the blunder with a different cartridge, contact Member Care through telephone or online talk for help with the cartridge that is provoking the mistake.

Play out a Hard Reset on the machine. If this doesn't help, continue to

If the Cricut keeps on demonstrating the blunder message or demonstrates the mistake message with various cartridges, if you don't mind contact Member Care through one of the alternatives beneath for further help.

Cricut Expression 2

Blunder Message when the cartridge is embedded, Machine doesn't understand cartridges

Expel the cartridge and after that set it back in the Expression 2. If the blunder message comes up, or the machine generally doesn't peruse the cartridge, continue to 2.

Attempt another cartridge in the machine. If this cartridge works, it would be ideal if you contact Member Care for help with the cartridge that isn't working. If the issue happens with all cartridges, it would be ideal if you contact Member Care by means of telephone or online talk for further help.

Cricut Imagine

The machine won't read "heritage" cartridges, or won't perceive Imagine cartridges

"Update Machine" message when embeddings cartridges

The machine won't read "heritage" cartridges, or won't perceive Imagine Cartridges

Attempt another cartridge in the machine. If the subsequent cartridge works in the machine, contact Member Care through one of the alternatives beneath for help with the first cartridge that wasn't working. If the subsequent cartridge likewise doesn't work, it would be ideal if you contact Member Care through one of the alternatives underneath for help.

"Update Machine" message when embeddings cartridges

PRACTICAL EXAMPLES AND STRATEGIES FOR EVERY KIND OF PROJECT

What appeared to be so natural for reasons unknown never was. I never at any point got into entangled undertakings like print and cut, I extremely simply needed to cut vinyl, and for reasons unknown, it just never worked right the first run through. That electronic slicing machine went to a companion or a relative, never to be utilized again.

Then I evaluated the Cricut Explore Air. Furthermore, before I go any further, let me reveal to you how to say Cricut because as a novice to the specialty business, I actually called it Cri-Cut (like cry-cut) everlastingly feeling that it was some extravagant name that solitary use crafters realized how to articulate. It's most certainly not. You articulate it like cricket, the bug.

What's more, if you're somewhat more attentive than I was, you'll see there's charming little cricket recieving wires in the logo. I'm going to credit my idiocy to being pregnant and baby blues mind haze.

CRICUT PROJECTS TO MAKE WITH THE CRICUT MACHINE

Just in the event that you're as terrified of utilizing an electronic cutting machine as I seemed to be, let me give you a little taste of what you can make with it. These tasks are, for the most part, totally different, and all made with the Cricut Explore Air. What's more, I can hardly wait to attempt every one of them!

Here are only a couple of different sorts of things you can do! I likewise incorporated some model Cricut ventures you can make with the Cricut Explore Air from a portion of my preferred shrewd companions!

#1 – CUT PAPER PRODUCTS WITH THE CRICUT EXPLORE AIR

You can go as straightforward or as mind boggling as you need – simply take a gander at this perplexing design from my companion Cori at Hey, Let's Make Stuff!

You can either design your own thing in Cricut Design Space, use designs as of now there, or simply use designs officially made for you in Cricut Design Space!

Sewing Star Pallet Sign

DIY Lunch Notes by Jen Goode

Cut Letter with your Cricut Explore

Straightforward Ice Cream Cone Shirt

The most effective method to Cut Chipboard and wood with the Cricut Explore

Gold Foil Vinyl Wood Teepee

The most effective method to utilize Cricut Design Space on your Ipad and Phone

Utilizing the Cricut Design Space App is an incredible method to make the most of your machine, you can your entrance your pictures, prepared to cut undertakings, and the best part is that you DON'T require web!

If you are as of now acquainted with the Desktop adaptation of Cricut Design Space, you will discover this application exceptionally simple to explore. Simply make a plunge, tap, investigate, and don't be apprehensive, your Phone or Ipad won't detonate!

Then again, if you have no experience at all, this is the best spot for you to be, this book will take you on each and every little symbol the App has.

I comprehend that learning another aptitude can be a bit of baffling at the occasions, however when you take the time and are tolerance with it, you can turn into a specialist.

Since the vast majority of the screen captures you will see next are taken from my iPad, I need to bring up the differences you will discover between the Ipad and Iphone adaptation.

Is there any difference between Design Space App for iPhone and iPad? Fortunate for you and me there's not by any stretch of the imagination a major difference between these two choices. Would you be able to envision attempting to learn two different applications?

The main little difference between the application for Iphone and Ipad is the SPACE MANAGEMENT.

You will see this first on the top board where it deal (Home – Canvas – Make) on the iPad you will consistently observe the names, yet on the telephone, now and again, you will see a square shape isolated in three equivalent amounts of. Be that as it may, the two of them speak to something very similar.

Something to remember too is that the vast majority of the occasions when you tap on something the menus are long, so with the telephone you should slide them to one side and appropriate to see every one of the choices – now and then with the iPad as well.

Additionally, since space is so restricted, on your telephone the layers catch will be deactivated different the occasions when you tap on different highlights. On the iPad you can leave the layers catch noticeable at unsurpassed.

Understanding the Methodology of this instructional exercise

I think the most ideal approach to learn is by tracking with the way so proceed and – in the wake of getting some espresso/or tea obviously – and open your application from your iPhone or Ipad.

Each time you open your application just because you will be in the home area, from here you will almost certainly pick a prepared to cut venture, pictures and additionally Create a New Project.

When you tap on New Project – the blue square – you will be on the CANVAS AREA. This is where we are going to put the greater part of our endeavors to learn.

I accept that the most ideal approach to learn and ace Cricut Design Space is from the earliest starting point! When you have a reasonable idea of what each symbol and board is for, then you can genuinely dive in and begin investigating further and further.

Here and there we rush to hop from task to extend – Hey That's alright as well! BTDT – But I believe that knowing your work zone will assist you with taking your inventiveness in an unheard of level.

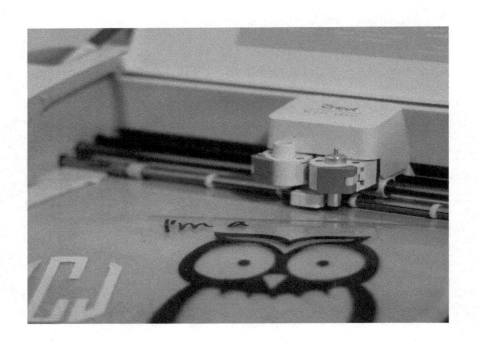

To make this simple for you I have separated the design region in three different segments. Top Panel (purple) Canvas Area (green/Bottom Panel (pink)

Is it true that you are prepared to handle each board/segment and see what happens when you tap any of the choices accessible?

Top Panel

This board enables you to explore from the Canvas to your profile, ventures, and it likewise enables you to extend the Canvas Space to the maximum.

a. Profile Picture – Settings

When you tap on your profile picture, a menu will slide open with two or three settings. From here you can set up your machine and furthermore observe a little application diagram of how the machine functions.

If you are anticipating utilizing Print then Cut choice with your Phone or iPad, this alignment guarantee will that everything will go easily.

There are different alternatives here that I prescribe you to see, I won't broadly expound on them because I wan to concentrate on the designs part of the application.

b. Spare

This alternative will actuate after you've set one component on your canvas region.

I suggest you spare your venture as you go, because, regardless of whether you are working from your gadget and the cloud you can run out battery, your application can crash and if that occurs, there goes your diligent work with it!

c. Home/Canvas/Make

These catches are a type of short code and they speak to the different perspectives you will have while utilizing the application. The darker region speaks to your present area.

Home will take you directly toward the start. If you needed to supplant your present undertaking and include another one tap here.

Canvas: is where you design and sort out a task before you cut it.

Make: tap here if you need to cut your undertaking. First you have to Tap make it on the Bottom Panel.

d. Extend

There are minutes, particularly when you are dealing with a little gadget, that you will need to see your design with ZERO diversions.

When you tap on this choice the Canvas Area will grow and every single other menu will be covered up. To return to your ordinary view, tap here.

Canvas Area

The Canvas region is the place the majority of the enchantment occurs! This is the place you play with your designs, get innovative, and finish things up before you cut them.

a. Estimations

The canvas region is separated by a lattice!

I think this element is extraordinary, because each and every square you see on the Grid encourages you to envision the cutting mat.

You can change the estimations from creeps to cm and turn the lattice on and off when you tap on the settings symbol situated on the base board of the application.

b. Determination

Whenever you select at least one layers, the determination is blue in shading and you can modify your choice from the majority of the 4 corners.

The red x, is for erasing the layers. The correct upper corner will enable you to pivot the picture. In spite of the fact that if you need a specific edge I prescribe you to utilize the pivot instrument situated in the base board when tapping the symbol Edit.

The little lock keeps the size corresponding when you increment or abatement the size of your layer with the lower right catch of the choice. By tapping on it, you are presently ready to have different extents.

There's additionally a fifth alternative between the lock and the size choice. When you tap on it and drag your design you can see it from different edges. I think this is valuable if you need to find in a 3D point of view (Specially if you have the camera choice initiated). When you let go, the determination will return to its unique structure

Savvy – Hand Gestures

Since we are working with innovation obviously we will be utilizing our fingers a great deal.

It's an extraordinary thought for you to see everything you can do with the tip of your fingers!

There are six signals you can use inside the application:

Tap: utilize a solitary tap to choose a picture or layer (likewise to choose any menu choices)

Swipe: if you have to choose more than one picture, simply swipe your finger on your screen to choose every one of the ones you need.

Tap and hold: You can choose a picture individually also. Complete an increasingly drawn out tap and after that select another design by doing likewise. To expel the determination, simply complete a solitary tap on the canvas territory.

Two Finger swipe: if you have to move around the canvas, you have to utilize 2 fingers simultaneously. Other shrewd you would do motion #2 (Swipe)

Twofold Tap: twofold tap to auto-zoom and see the majority of the components and designs you have on the canvas zone.

Squeeze Zoom: zoom in and out by utilizing your thumb and forefinger.

Base Panel

You folks.... .We are entering profound waters now, and there is no returning!

The base board may feel to you like be the most testing one because basically everything is done from here.

On the Cricut Design Space Desktop form the majority of the choices are isolated in three boards; yet on the application, they are for the most part hanging out together at base, while you become accustomed to it you may get disappointed attempting to discover the choice you need.

Each time you tap on one of the choices; the symbol itself will turn green and the alternatives of that instrument will either take you to another window or will slide open in a white menu simply like I show you on the screen capture directly above.

Note: contingent upon the size of your gadget, with the goal for you to see the majority of the choices of the menu, you should look over every menu to one side and right.

You can just utilize one choice at the time, aside from with the Layers choice, This one can be dynamic consistently. In any case, when the application on you iPhone, the layers board will move toward becoming deactivated all the time.

This application is extremely strong, and It has the greater part of the things that the Desktop form has. Toward the finish of this post, there is a rundown of the things that this application doesn't have.

a. Include Image

Pictures are immaculate when you are assembling your very own undertakings; with them, you can include an additional touch and character to your artworks.

You can look by catchphrase, classes, or cartridges. You can discover pictures you have recently transferred to your PC or your gadget.

Cartridges are a lot of pictures that you have to buy independently. Some of them accompany Cricut Access, and some not. The ones that are not accessible for Cricut Access are authorized brands, for example, Disney, Sesame Street, Hello Kitty, and so on.

Cricut has FREE pictures to cut each week. You can discover them when you tap on Categories.

If you will be looking an activities in the cloud the you would require web; however if you are simply going to utilize pictures you have on your gadget, or apparatuses from the application itself you can work with no web association.

Cool Right?

b. Include Text

Whenever you need to type on the Canvas Area, you should tap on Text.

After you tap you will be incited to pick the textual style you need to work with, and then a little box will show up on the canvas zone for you to type in your content.

c. Include Shapes

Having the option to utilize shapes, it's significant! With them, you can make straightforward, less perplexing, yet at the same time beautiful tasks.

There're are 9 shapes you can look over:

Square

Triangle

Pentagon

Hexagon

Star

Octagon

Heart

The principal alternative isn't a shape, however an astounding and useful asset called Score Line. With this alternative, you can make overlap and score your materials.

If you need to make boxes or love everything about card making, the Score Line will be your closest companion!

d. Transfer

With this alternative, you can transfer your very own records, and pictures that you need to cut. When you Tap on this choice, you will have the choice to pick the area of your photograph, or even take one. The web is load up with them, and there are huge amounts of bloggers that make extends for nothing. Truth be told I am one of them

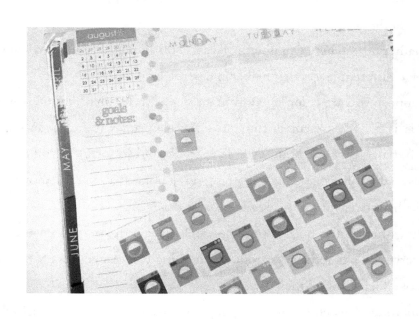

If you have no clue where to discover pictures or cut documents, I have a developing library that you can approach when you buy in to my bulletin and become a daydreamer!

e. Activities

The activities boards is a substantial one! From here you can absolutely change your design into a totally different one.

A portion of the choices here might befuddle you from the start, yet as I generally state; don't thump it until you've attempted it!

Gathering – Ungroup

Gathering: tap here to gathering layers. This setting is valuable when you have different layers that make up a perplexing design.

Suppose you are chipping away at an elephant. In all likelihood – and if this is a SVG or cut document – the elephant will be made out of different layers (the body, eyes, legs, trunk, and so forth). If you need to fuse, additional shapes, and content; no doubt is that you will move your elephant over the canvas region a great deal.

By gathering the majority of the elephant layers, you can ensure that everything will remain sort out and nothing will escape place when you move them around then canvas.

Ungroup: This choice will ungroup any assembled layers you select on the canvas region or layers board. This is valuable when you have to alter – size, kind of textual style, and so on – a specific component or layer from the gathering.

Join – Detach

This works like gathering layers; however it's all the more dominant.

When you select the two shapes and tap on append, the two layers will have now a similar shading – shading is dictated by the layer that is on the back – This connection will stay set up, even after I send my task to be cut.

If you want to separate your layers, select them again and tap on, withdraw

Weld

The welding instrument enables you to join to shapes in one.

When I chose the two shapes and tapped on weld, you can see that I made an entirely different shape. The shading is controlled by the layer that is on the back, that is the reason the new shape is pink in shading

Cut

The cut instrument is impeccable to remove shapes, content, and different components, from another designs.

When I chose the two shapes and tapped on cut. You can see that the first record got all cut up. To demonstrate to you what the last item was, I reordered the cut outcome and the isolated the majority of the pieces that came about because of cutting.

Level – Unflatten

This layer is an additional help for the Print and Cut layer characteristic. When you change the credit from slice to print, that applies to only one layer. Yet, imagine a scenario in which you simply need to do it to numerous shapes at the time.

When you are finished with your designed (you can just unflatten or turn around before leaving your undertaking), select the layers you need to print together all in all, and afterward, tap on level.

On this case, the component was changed over to print and cut. That is the reason it's not demonstrating a dark edge – where the cutting edge will experience – any longer.

Copy

This choice will copy any layers or designs you have chosen on the layers board or canvas region.

This is exceptionally valuable because you don't need to reproduce the design, starting with no outside help. It resembles duplicating and glue.

Shroud Contour

For this model, I consolidated the first design fit as a fiddle with the weld device. Then I composed the word form and cut it against the new shape. The Contour apparatus enables you to shroud undesirable bits of a design, and it may be initiated when a shape or design has components that can be forgotten about.

When you tap on form, another window will spring up with the majority of the pieces on the design that can be cut of on the left.

For this specific realistic, I concealed the inward circles of the two letters O and the internal piece of the letter R.

Detach Letters

This alternative is accessible for content layers. Fundamentally when you select content and tap on Isolate Layers, you will probably alter each and every letter without anyone else.

The work area form has further developed choices for content, yet this a decent begin. Possibly one they will include different choices.

f. Alter Menu

The alter menu enables you to modify your content significantly further. You can likewise adjust, mastermind, and sort out the majority of the component you have on the canvas territory.

We should see all off the things you can achieve when you tap on this menu.

When you tap on this catch, you can choose any text style you need to use for your undertakings. You can channel them and quest for them on the highest point of window.

If you have Cricut Access, you can utilize any of the considerable number of text styles that have somewhat green A toward the start of the textual style title.

When you pick your text style, you have the alternatives to change its style.

These are the most widely recognized alternatives:

– Regular: This is the default setting. What's more, it wont change the presence of your textual style

– Bold: It will make the text style thicker .

– Italic: It will tilt the textual style to one side.

– Bold italic: it will make the textual style thicker and tilt to one side.

In some cases, the textual style itself will have pretty much choices, The one I utilized for this Screenshot had far more alternatives.

Tip: If you are utilizing Cricut text styles, you will see that with some of them, you can likewise utilize the compose choice.

Arrangement

This arrangement is selective for content. It's incredible for you to compose passages and lines of content.

These are the alternatives you have:

31

– Left: Align a passage to one side

– Center: Align a passage to the inside

– Right: Align a passage to one side.

Size, Letter, and Line Space

I can't express enough how AMAZING these choices are. Uncommonly the letter separating.

Text dimension: You can transform it physically from here. I regularly simply alter the size of my textual styles from the canvas region.

Letter Space: There are text styles that have a major hole between each letter. This alternative will enable you to diminish the space between letters in all respects effectively. It's genuinely a distinct advantage.

Line Space: this alternative will handle the space between lines in a section. This is valuable because now and then I am compelled to make a solitary lines of content because I am not content with the dividing between lines.

Size

All that you make or type on the Cricut Design Space canvas has a size. You can modify the size from the component in self (when you tap on it). Be that as it may, if you need a component to be an accurate estimation, this choice will enable you to do as such.

Something significant is the little lock on that estimation. When you increment or lessen the size of a picture, the extents are constantly bolted. By tapping on the little lock, you are telling the application that you would prefer not to keep similar extents.

Turn

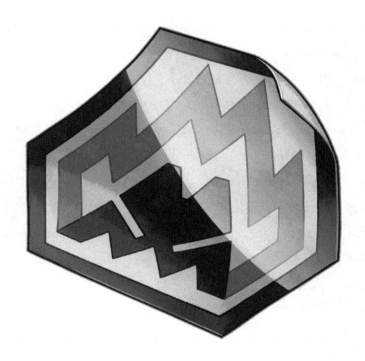

Much the same as size, pivoting a component is something you can do in all respects effectively from the canvas region. Notwithstanding, there are designs that should be pivoted on a specific point. If that is the situation for you, I really prescribe you to utilize this capacity. Else, you will invest so much energy battling to get a component calculated the manner in which you need it to be.

Flip

If you have to mirror any of your designs on the Cricut Design Space, this is an incredible method to do it.

There are 2 alternatives:

– Flip Horizontal: This will mirror your picture or design on a level plane. Similar to a mirror; It's valuable when you are attempting to make left and right designs. Model: You are making a few wings, or simply have the left wing. With this, you can reorder that equivalent wing and the flip it. Presently you have both!

– Flip Vertical: This is will flip your designs vertically. Sort of like you would see your appearance on water. If you need to make a shadow impact, this choice would be extraordinary for you.

Position

This case demonstrates to you where your components are on the canvas region when you tap on a specific design.

You can move your components around by specifying where you need that component to be situated on the canvas zones. It's exceptionally valuable; however an it's a further developed instrument.

I, for one, don't utilize it that much. I can show signs of improvement with the arrangement devices I am going to make reference to.

Mastermind

Something truly cut about this capacity is that the program will recognize what component is on the front or back and, and when you select it, Design space will actuate the accessible choices for that specific component. Cool right?

These are the choices you get:

– Send to back: This will move the chose component right to the back.

– Move Backward: This alternative will move chosen the component only one stage back. S.o if you have a three component design. It will resemble the cheddar in a cheddar sandwich.

– Move Forward: This choice will move the component only one stage forward. Ordinarily, you would utilize this choice when you have at least 4 components you have to sort out.

– Sent to front: This choice will move the chose component right to the front.

Arrangement

This capacity enables you to adjust the majority of your designs, and it's enacted when select at least 2 components.

– Center: This choices is an exceptionally cool one. When you tap on focus, you are focusing, both vertically and on a level plane; one design against another. This is exceptionally valuable when you need to focus content with a shape like a square or star.

– Align Left: When utilizing this setting, the majority of your components will be adjusted to one side. The uttermost component to one side will direct where the majority of different components will move.

– Align Center: This choice will adjust your components evenly. This will totally focus content and pictures.

— Align Right: When utilizing this setting, the majority of your components will be adjusted to one side. The farthest component to the correct will manage where the majority of different components will move.

— Align Top: This choice will adjust the majority of your chose designs to the top. The uttermost component to the top will direct where the majority of different components will move.

— Align Middle: This alternative will adjust your components vertically. It's valuable when you are working with sections , nd you need them sorted out and adjusted.

— Align Bottom: This alternative will adjust the majority of your chose designs to the base. The uttermost component to the base will direct where the majority of different components will move.

If you need a similar separating between components, it's very tedious to do everything all alone, and it's not 100% right. The appropriate catch will enable you to out with that. For it to be initiated, you should have in any event three components chose.

— Distribute Horizontally: This catch will disperse the components evenly. The uttermost left and right designs will decide the length of the dissemination. This implies the components that are in the inside will be dispersed between the uttermost left and right designs.

ALL YOU NEED TO KNOW TO BECOME A PROFESSIONAL

Did you get a Cricut as of late? If you've ended up considering how to utilize a Cricut, which tangle to utilize and how to finish your first task, this post is for you!

I'll walk you through everything from opening your container, and buying the correct supplies to finishing your absolute first task!

Would it be a good idea for me to Buy A Cricut Maker?

All things considered, first of all… here's a little foundation on the Cricut Maker. The Cricut Maker is an electronic cutting machine (additionally called an art plotter or bite the dust cutting machine). You can consider it like a printer; you make a picture or design on your PC, cell phone, or tablet, and after that send it to the machine. Then again, actually as opposed to printing your design, the Maker removes it of whatever material you need! (The Maker can cut more than 100 different materials! Here's a rundown of 100+ materials that a Cricut Maker can cut.)

The Cricut Maker is extraordinary for crafters, quilters, sewers, DIYers, and any other person with an inventive streak! It has a versatile apparatus framework that enables you to switch among cutting edges and extras so you can do any sort of task. Need to cut sewing examples and texture? Change to the revolving cutting edge. Need to cut balsa wood or calfskin? Change to the knife cutting edge. Need to draw something, or add scoring lines to your undertaking? The Cricut pen and scoring wheel are immaculate! Regardless of what kind of undertaking you need to do, the Cricut Maker can deal with it!

What's more, to demonstrate you exactly that it is so natural to make amazing things with a Cricut Maker, I have a too straightforward cowhide bow venture instructional exercise toward the finish of this post. It'll take you under 10 minutes! I additionally made a fast video that strolls you through the whole starting arrangement your Maker machine, including making your first venture: an adorable welcome card. Look at it to see exactly that it is so natural to utilize the machine!

Will I utilize the machine enough to justify the cost?

This is the issue I hear regularly, and it's absolutely reasonable! The Cricut Maker is typically $399.99 (however you can generally discover it at a bargain), which is surely a speculation. Nobody needs to spend that sort of money on something that will get utilized each day for a month and afterward simply lounge around social occasion dust!

However, I wouldn't stress over that with the Cricut Maker; there are SO MANY different things you can do with it. I don't think you'll ever get exhausted. I've had my Cricut machines throughout recent years despite everything I use them consistently! If you're searching for task thoughts, I have a Pinterest board loaded up with Cricut ventures, and here's a rundown of more than 100 art and DIY ventures you can make with a Cricut machine.

What additional items do I have to utilize the machine, and how costly will it be?

The Cricut Maker accompanies completely all that you have to utilize the machine directly in the container! It even has test materials so you can make your absolute first venture immediately!

All things considered, probably the coolest thing about the Maker is that is has a versatile instrument framework which enables you to change out the sharp edges and devices to do different kinds of activities. The Maker accompanies a fine-point sharp edge (the standard edge for everything from paper to card stock), a fine-point pen for illustration, and a rotational edge for cutting texture. It likewise accompanies a LightGrip tangle (for paper and so forth.) and a FabricGrip tangle for cutting texture with the rotational sharp edge. Between those two cutting edges and those two mats, you can cut pretty much anything you need. You could utilize your Maker each and every day with simply the things that come in the container for always, and you'd never get exhausted!

Obviously, there are extras and additional items you can purchase for your machine if you need. Cricut is continually turning out with new apparatuses and sharp edges; however the most well-known additional items for a Maker are:

The knife edge (about $45, except if you discover it at a bargain): enables you to cut thicker materials like balsa wood or calfskin

The scoring wheels (about $40, except if you discover them on special): permits you make fresh, clean score lines in your activities

Extra pens or markers (about $12 for a 5-pack, except if you discover them at a bargain): comes in huge amounts of hues and thicknesses, including metallics, sparkles, fine point, and calligraphy pens

The other spot you could spend extra cash if you need to is in the Cricut picture and text styles library. It is allowed to utilize Cricut Design Space (their online design programming), and they have huge amounts of pictures and textual styles that you can use for nothing. What's more, obviously, you can generally transfer your very own pictures and utilize those.

If you would prefer not to utilize your very own pictures, the library has more than 50,000 pictures, several text styles, huge amounts of prepared to-make ventures, authorized characters, and so on that you can use for your tasks. What's more, extremely, a LOT of it is free! In any case, for certain things, you need to buy the picture or text styles before you can utilize them in your activities. You can purchase pictures exclusively (normally about $0.99) or in cartridges or "sets" (more often than not about $5 to $30), and once you've gotten them you can utilize them in a boundless number of tasks.

You can likewise pursue Cricut Access, which is their month to month membership which gives you access to more than 50,000 pictures and 400 textual styles, in addition to a 10% markdown on some other Cricut items! Cricut Access memberships are $7.99/month or $9.99/month for their Premium enrollment, which gives you free delivering and up to half off authorized text styles, pictures, and prepared to-make extends (the authorized stuff like Disney characters and so on is excluded in the 50,000 free pictures because, well, it's authorized!)

What materials would i be able to cut?

Pretty much anything you need! The Cricut Maker can slice materials up to 2.4mm thick, and it can cut stuff as slight and fragile as tissue paper. Here's a rundown of 100+ materials that a Cricut Maker can cut.

What sorts of texture would i be able to cut, and do I need a supporter? Indeed, I simply shared a rundown of 100+ materials a Cricut can cut; however, texture is somewhat exceptional and gets its own different segment!

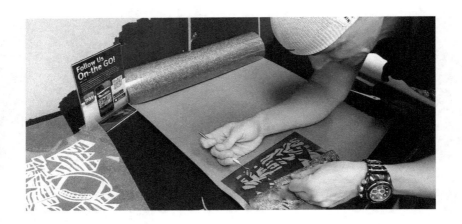

Perhaps the coolest thing about the Maker is that it enables you to cut texture without a supporter when you utilize the turning edge! Past adaptations of the Cricut machines had the option to cut texture with the normal fine-point edge; however you needed to stiffen it up first by putting interfacing on the back of the texture. That is fine and all, yet now and again you don't need interfacing on the back of your task, which is the reason the revolving sharp edge is great. (Furthermore, the fine-point sharp edge is positively ready to cut texture; however the edges of the cuts aren't really excessively perfect and fresh... the revolving cutting edge completes a MUCH better activity!)

The Maker can cut practically any texture, from sensitive textures like tulle and ribbon to substantial textures like denim, sailcloth, and burlap. It can likewise cut "claim to fame" textures like sequined textures, texture with sparkle on it, calfskin, fake hide, and even blanket batting. When you utilize the rotating cutting edge to cut texture, you needn't bother with a supporter; you can put the texture straightforwardly onto the FabricGrip tangle and cut it without anyone else. Or on the other hand, if you need a support on your texture, don't hesitate to connect the sponsorship before you cut; the turning edge can deal with the two layers with no issue! Truth be told, the Maker can slice up to three layers of texture simultaneously, which is magnificent for things like blanket making or texture ventures with numerous pieces in a similar shape.

Will it be simple for me to get familiar with the product and use it to design my own venture or prepare to-make ventures?

That's right, I suspect as much! I really imagine that Cricut Design Space is quite natural, regardless of whether you're not by any means well informed. Cricut has a little walkthrough instructional exercise that you experience when you initially set up your machine, and it completes a truly great job of demonstrating to you the nuts and bolts of Design Space (in any event, enough to make any of the prepared to-make extends in the Cricut library). Also, if you need to design your very own ventures, I have a lot of well ordered instructional exercises on the most proficient method to utilize a Cricutthat you can look at.

If you're still somewhat apprehensive, I made a video that strolls you through the whole introductory arrangement of your Cricut Maker, including making your absolute first undertaking! It tells you the best way to utilize the fundamental elements of Design Space to make a basic welcome card.

What sorts of specialties and DIY undertakings would i be able to make? As far as possible, here is your creative mind! You can make basically anything from welcome cards and paper ventures to home stylistic theme to wedding/party/occasion enrichments to attire and blankets. There are such a large number of different things you can make that I'd always be unable to show them all. Be that as it may, here is a rundown of 100+ specialties and DIY ventures you can make with a Cricut, and here is my Pinterest board brimming with Cricut venture thoughts; those will at any rate kick you off!

Would i be able to utilize my old cartridges?

The first Cricut machines utilized physical plastic cartridges that you could embed into the machine itself to access picture content. The physical cartridges have been resigned, and now Cricut has computerized cartridges (essentially a "picture set" of related pictures accessible in the Cricut library).

Be that as it may, don't stress! If you have physical cartridges from a past Cricut machine, you can absolutely still utilize those pictures! You can connect your physical cartridge to the advanced form in Cricut Design Space, and afterward, you can utilize the computerized variant of the majority of your pictures whenever you need.

Would i be able to transfer my very own pictures?

That's right! Here is a well ordered instructional exercise telling you the best way to transfer your very own pictures to Cricut Design Space. You can transfer fundamental pictures like a jpeg or png, or you can transfer a vector record if you have a picture that has numerous layers. Design Space supports transfer of the accompanying document types:

jpg

gif

png

bmp

svg

dxf

If you have questions that weren't replied in this post, don't hesitate to email me and ask them! I'm constantly glad to help!

As guaranteed, here is a fast instructional exercise on making calfskin bows with a Cricut Maker. This undertaking requires a Cricut Maker, the knife cutting edge, a StrongGrip tangle, and a bit of calfskin.

Begin by opening up this calfskin bow venture in Cricut Design Space. If you click the green Make It catch, the bow is now measured to be 1" tall and about 2.5" wide. If you need to change the size or make various duplicates, click the Customize catch to open the undertaking in Design Space.

Select "Book of clothing Leather" in the materials segment, and the product will instruct you to stack the knife edge in your Maker. Open Clamp B, expel the fine-point sharp edge and introduce the knife edge, so the apparatuses on the cutting edge meet with the riggings in the machine. Close the clasp.

Spot your calfskin on the StrongGrip tangle, face up, then burden the tangle into the machine. Press the glimmering Go catch, and the machine will begin to cut! (If this is the first occasion when you've utilized your knife cutting edge, the product will walk you through adjusting the knife sharp edge, so you get exact cuts.)

After the machine gets done with writing, it will request that you check the slice to ensure it's gone right through the material. Ensure you don't empty the tangle first! Simply twist the tangle somewhat directly at the edge of a cut, and if you can see right through the material to the tangle underneath, then you're ready. If it didn't carve entirely through, press the Go catch again to make it cut once again.

What Comes with the Cricut Maker?

Cricut Maker with Fine Point Blade

We should Get Started Box (Included URL for arrangement)

Welcome Book and Rotary Blade

Fine Point Pen

Guarantee

USB Cord and Power Cord

A Piece of Cardstock and Fabric (for your first task)

12 x 12 Light Grip and Fabric Grip Mat

50 Free Ready-to-Make Projects, Including 25 Sewing Patterns

Free Trial Membership to Cricut Access™ (for new endorsers)

Which Cricut Mat Should I Use?

Blue Light Grip Mat

This tangle is perfect for light weight materials. It gives enough hold to keep the material set up during slicing yet enables it to be effectively evacuated without tearing.

Printer Paper, Vellum, Light Cardstock, Construction Paper, Vinyl and Cardstock

Green Standard Mat

The standard tangle is perfect for the amplest assortment of materials. It gives a more grounded grasp which enables it to immovably hold heavier materials set up with simple.

Designed Paper, Vinyl, Iron-On, Cardstock, Embossed Cardstock, Heavey Cardstock

Purple Strong Grip Mat

The most grounded of the Cricut mats, this tangle is ideal for thick and heavyweight materials. It highlights twofold life glue innovation, which enables it to effectively grasp onto increasingly strong materials and hold them set up all through the cutting procedure.

Forte Cardstock, Chipboard, Backed Fabrics, Leather, Magnet Sheet, and Felt

Pink Fabric Mat

The texture tangle is produced using higher-quality PVC to withstand expanded cutting weight. It includes a different glue than the other cutting mats settling on it the perfect decision for texture and th ideal counterpart for the Cricut Rotary Blade.

Silk, Canvas, Burlap, Cotton, and that's only the tip of the iceberg

The most effective method to Use A Cricut Mat

To utilize the glue Cricut cutting mat, expel the unmistakable defensive liner. Spot it to the side while the tangle is being used and place it back on the tangle once you have completed the process of utilizing it.

Spot the material you are working with (right side up) inside the 12" x 12" matrix, ensuring that the whole material has clung to the tangle completley.

Which Cricut Accessories Do I Need To Get Started Crafting?

I suggest obtaining an Essential Tool Set before you start creating! This will have the majority of the things you have to make stunning tasks rapidly and effectively!

This instrument set incorporates:

Invert Tweezers to lift and verify sensitive materials

Weeder enables you to expel little negative pieces from the design

Scissors with Protective Cover

Calculated Spatula to lift materials from the tangle without bowing them

Scrubber to polish materials and clean cutting mats

Scoring Stylus to make crease lines on cards

12" Wide Material Trimmer to precisely cut Vinyl, Iron-On, and Cardstock

Swap Blades for Trimmer

Scoring Blade for Trimmer to add scoring lines to different tasks

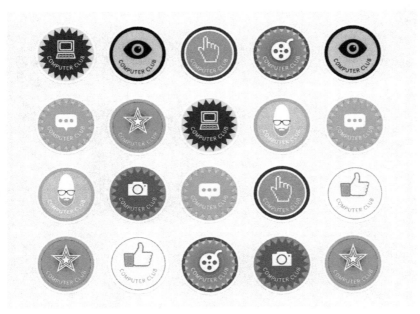

What Supplies Should I Purchase?

I prescribe obtaining a wide range of materials so you can get familiar with the wide assortment of materials that your Cricut Maker is equipped for cutting. The following are a couple of the materials I would prescribe acquiring!

Removable Vinyl Variety Pack 12 x 12

Move Tape

Ordinary Iron-On Rainbow Sampler

Cardstock Rainbow Sampler 12 x 24

Texture Sampler Pack

Felt Sampler Pack

5 Pen Variety Pack

Knife Blade

Scoring Wheels

What's the Difference among Vinyl and Iron-On?

There are two different kinds of Vinyl, Adhesive vinyl which has a sticky support and is connected with weight and Iron-On (additionally alluded to as Heat Transfer Vinyl) which has a paste backing that is actuated by warmth.

Iron-On and Heat Transfer Vinyl

Iron-On is perfect for ventures that can withstand heat. The surface ought to be smooth and ready to have an iron connected to it. Instances of appropriate materials are:

Shirts

Texture

Cushions

Wood

Cardstock

Canvas Tote Bags

Iron-On has a paste backing that clings to a surface once it's been initiated by warmed. YOu can apply Iron-On with an iron, EasyPress or Heat Press. You can peruse progressively about the Easy Press here.

A reasonable defensive liner is situated over the Iron-On, this enables the vinyl to be warmed without being harmed and is stripped far from the design once it has clung to the material. Iron-On should be cut with the liner side (really side) confronting downwards and any content or pictures ought to be turned around or reflected.

Glue Vinyl

Vinyl is perfect for surfaces that are hard just as smooth. Instances of things that can have vinyl concerned them are mugs, wood, dividers, mirrors, and glass. It tends to be cut with the correct side confronting upwards and the liner confronting downwards towards the Cricut tangle.

How Do I Clean My Cricut Mats and Fabric Mat?

To clean the Cricut Light, Standard and Strong Grip Mats absorb the tangle warm foamy water. Delicately perfect any remaining buildup with Non-Alcohol Baby Wipes. Utilize your Scraper to expel any difficult bits of buildup.

To clean the pink Cricut Fabric Grip tangle basically expel any stray strings with a lot of invert tweezers. The glue is different on this tangle and ought not be washed!

HOW TO TURN YOUR CREATIVITY INTO AN AMAZING BUSINESS

Neighborhood deals can be separated into two sections, business to business (B2B) and business to client (B2C). If you choose to be a neighborhood merchant, it's ideal to pick between one of these two fragments.

These two gatherings don't have much cover in the things they buy, or where you can market to them. The reasonable entrepreneur won't squander their time pursuing leads and tossing showcasing cash at customers they aren't arrangement to help.

Business to Business –

Volume Sales - The objective here is to utilize the productivity of creating in bigger numbers to drive the cost you pay per thing down. The bigger the generation run, the lower your expense for item and time per unit created. This is the hardest work to get into for another Cricut or Silhouette based business. The open doors are less, and the customer desires are higher.

Models:

An agreement with the neighborhood government or school to deliver shirts or signage.

Yearly occasion signage and promoting, for example, signage and shirts for the Susan G. Komen Foundation

Aces –

Regularly, legally binding work can be finished in a solitary session. This implies you can buy from sellers in mass, enabling you to arrange lower material expenses. You will likewise have less exchanging between vinyl hues or product offerings, which means you can accomplish more in less time. This leaves you with more opportunity for different undertakings or showcasing endeavors.

Cons –

It will be hard to get one of these agreements. As a matter of fact, I haven't attempted. It is sensible to expect that these open doors in your locale are now being served by another person. If they aren't, jump at the opportunity.

Custom Work – Custom work for business clients, can be an incredible gig with enormous upside. Organizations are happy to pay as much as possible for quality, solid work. You can work with organizations to help make a brand character, make mindfulness, and make special promotions.

Models:

If a business is simply beginning, you can offer a business dispatch starter pack. At least, you ought to incorporate logo design, signage for a retail front, and establishment.

You can likewise offer organization marked swag like shirts, cups, or mugs as an extra. Every one of these administrations can be independent for new or existing organizations.

Signage, for example, sandwich sheets or yard signs.

Stars –

You are making associations with developing organizations. After your first effective exchange, you become their place of contact for future business marking, decals, mindfulness materials, and even visual depiction. This relationship can pay future profits.

Business customers accompany numerous open doors for up selling. More often than not, it is a success win for both of you.

Cons –

It very well may be difficult to discover new, quality leads. For most existing organizations, they as of now have a sign organization they trust. All things considered, they needed to get their unique signs some place, isn't that so?

Entrepreneurs will, in general, be shrewd, with elevated requirements and a solid feeling of what is a suitable cost for your administration. Try not to be shocked or insulted if they get various offers and arrange cost before tolerating your offer.

Business to Customer–

Volume Sales - These standards are equivalent to with business to business mass work, yet you're going to discover your clients in new places and have different contributions.

You will sell things that retail clients need to purchase. This incorporates one of a kind shirt, tumblers, espresso cups, or whatever else you can think of. The key is to have expansive intrigue, something you can create various with the desire that they will sell.

Models:

Leasing a space at a classical shopping center or art reasonable. Make sure to evaluate how much space you really need, the value per square foot, and the commission your landowner is requesting.

Become a seller at neighborhood occasions. For instance, my wife was a merchant at the Mutt Strut in Nashville, Tennessee this year.

Discover space in popup shops

Discover occasional occasions in your town that offer shabby or free retail space, similar to a rancher's market or occasion reasonable.

Go out business cards to neighborhood shops where you envision your items may sell well.

Aces –

Your imagination will be the driver of your deals. If you concoct a sharp thought with mass or specialty claim, and you are in the opportune spot to offer it, you will receive the benefits. Additionally, you get the opportunity to figure out what media and medium you work in. Shirts, mugs, or whatever else, the decision is yours.

Cons –

You'll require a retail space to offer your things. The spots with higher pedestrian activity will be progressively costly, yet pedestrian activity doesn't really rise to deals.

To be effective, you'll should be eager to explore different avenues regarding different areas and item contributions.

Custom Work –

Models:

One of a kind shirts for a wedding party

Divider decals with one of a kind statements and family names

Monograms for wine glasses or vehicle decals

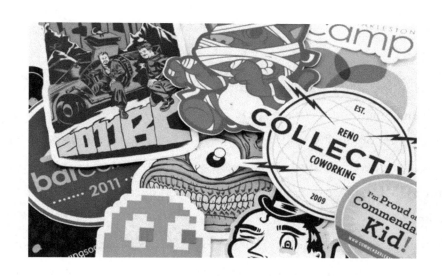

Experts –

Custom work for nearby clients has the most reduced startup cost of any of these procedures. If you can locate a solid seller who offers materials in little bunches, you can concede putting resources into vinyl until you secure a task.

You can likewise do the majority of your work from home, evading the need to put resources into a retail front or work space.

You will almost certainly charge a premium for your work. Retail clients pay the most astounding costs, and your design customization will raise the cost as well.

Cons –

Once more, leads will be difficult to get. Toward the start, verbal exchange might be the main device you have. You're going to need to concentrate on quality workmanship and reasonable valuing to get your underlying deals. If you have a touch of cash, you can kick begin the procedure by showcasing with a neighborhood Facebook promotion.

Selling Online

Concentrating on web based selling requires a higher specialized learning base, at the same time, as I can verify, you don't need to be a software engineer to make it work. You can profit with vinyl online by giving quality custom work, turning into a data center, or giving mass contributions. Once more, it's not prudent to attempt to do every one of the three.

Your time is best spent working in one of the three choices to start. In this way, if you choose to give custom work, don't likewise attempt to turn into a data center simultaneously. In the wake of building up your underlying balance and getting beneficial deals, you can anticipate how to utilize that cash for developing into different classifications.

Custom Work – This is the manner by which I got my begin. For the correct individual, I really accept this is an incredible method to the opening shot your Silhouette or Cricut vinyl business.

Through existing commercial centers or your own site, you can turn into the one they go to.

Models:

Existing sites that enable you to sell specially craft administrations. Etsy, Amazon Custom, and Amazon Handmade are the most notable. Different choices incorporate Artfire, DaWanda, Bonanza, Depop, and Tictail

Another alternative is to dispatch your very own site. An incredible case of this can be seen with A Great Impression. They propelled a rousing divider decal site, alongside a specially craft administration. You can get any decal, in any size you need from them.

Tip: I would suggest their procedure. Discover a specialty little enough you can contend inside, and offer hand crafts from that point.

Masters -

If you sell on a current stage, the startup expenses are exceptionally low. The minute you dispatch, you're contending in the worldwide marketplace. You approach a large number of potential clients.

Furthermore, one of a kind designs will enable you to charge an excellent rate. Nonetheless, online custom costs will, in general, be lower than a similar work done locally. It's an opportunity to clean up and expand your design range of abilities too.

Cons -

Access to the whole world additionally implies you are going up against anybody with a web association. Expanded challenge will prompt lower costs for your designs and difficulty getting occupations if you aren't intensely valued or offering an extraordinary design viewpoint.

Selling on the web implies you likewise need to learn coordination. You're going to need to get entered in with a transportation organization, make sense of pressing material, and calculate that cost your estimating. Volume Sales – The advantages of doing work in mass online are equivalent to neighborhood. By accomplishing more work without a moment's delay and diminishing the occasions we make switches between hues, designs, and product offerings, you're driving the expense per unit created down. You'll discover your clients through existing sites or by building up your own.

Models:

The greatest stages for mass design work are eBay and Amazon, in spite of the fact that Etsy has seen development in these sorts of offers in the course of the most recent three years. On these stages, you can sell window decals, moving expressions, divider specks, vehicle decals, shirts, and so on. Essentially, anything with an extreme interest that you can replicate various occasions after the underlying design.

Another alternative is to pick a specialty and offer a similar sort of work without anyone else site. Spotted Decals is an incredible case of this strategy. They are a little organization that works in divider specks just, nothing else. They are the expert when it comes to spotted decals. Because it is specialty and repeatable, the work should be possible in mass, and they face negligible challenge.

Geniuses -

You can begin to manufacture a genuine retail business selling this sort of work. After some time, you will most likely figure out what the interest for the designs you offer and plan generation ahead as needs be. This will build your productivity and lower the

You'll additionally be making more items. In all actuality, you will acquire less cash per deal; however this will allow you to purchase vinyl in mass at a diminished cost.

Cons -

You're going toward the world here. There's a huge amount of rivalry, so the edges will be lower, and quite possibly's somebody can undermine your little edges with phony or fake things anytime.

It's takes significant stage information to sell on the majority of the different commercial centers (eBay, Amazon, Etsy, and so on.).

Data Hub – Have you at any point visited a blog for guidance on the best way to utilize your machine or undertaking motivation? If you can dispatch a site and become the expert in the field, there's a chance to profit with your Silhouette Cameo or Cricut there as well.

Models - There are some extraordinary instances of web journals offering specialized expertise and task motivation with a specialty shaper. Some likewise couple their Cricut and Silhouette learning with a lifestyle blog.

Satisfaction's Life

Only a Girl and Her Blog

Cutting for Business

Ginger Snap Crafts

Lia Griffith

Salty Canary

CutCutCraft

Stars -

You're not making decals for clients any longer, and yourventures pursue your course of events. This implies you get the chance to be particular about the posts you take on, and the time you put into an undertaking. Additionally, you can express your inventiveness anyway you'd like and manufacture the group of spectators you need.

Cons -

How about we repeat, you're not making decals for clients any longer. This plan of action is totally different than the remainder of the choices I've spread out.

You can adapt your site with promotions, supported posts, offering an information item like a book for your devoted perusers, or a physical item. Be that as it may, regardless of which course you take, it's not as immediate, nor basic, as selling a decal.

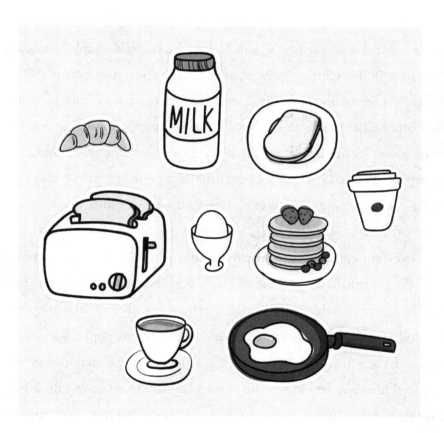

STEP BY STEP INSTRUCTIONS TO CUT PDF SEWING PATTERNS ON THE CRICUT MAKER

I'm infatuated with my new Cricut Maker! It's fast and simple to change over your PDF examples to be removed on this stunning new machine. Regardless of whether you don't have the Cricut Maker, you can utilize your other Cricut machines (Explore Air, and Explore Air2) to remove your paper example pieces as well! I utilize mine everything an opportunity to make my doll garments sewing quicker and increasingly exact. As a designer of doll garments PDF designs, this machine has made my activity speedier and simpler after a little set up regardless.

I got my Cricut Maker for Christmas. I've been utilizing cricut machines since they originally turned out and have possessed every single one that they have made. I think this Maker machine is a distinct advantage for the doll garments network, particularly if you sew for specialty fairs. I have a feeling that I've been hanging tight for it the majority of my "sewing" life. You would now be able to cut texture by essentially laying it on the tangle. There is no compelling reason to apply any stiffener so as to cut it with this phenomenal, new machine. The Cricut Maker is the main machine that has another rotational cutting sharp edge that was specifically made for texture. See progressively about this astounding machine here!

The Cricut Design Space library has many sewing designs for dolls. They cost about equivalent to the PDF designs you purchase from Oh Sew Kat! However, consider the possibility that don't care for those styles , r you need to make something other than what's expected. I've assembled this essential instructional exercise to walk you through the means of how to cut your Oh Sew Kat! PDF designs on your Cricut Maker machine (or cut your paper designs on other cricut machines-likewise a help!) There are numerous approaches to do this, however ,this is the strategy I have utilized , nd once you do it more than once, it's extremely quite speedy!

If you don't mind NOTE: Sharing a SVG record (on the web or face to face) you make from a PDF Pattern you acquired is equivalent to sharing the example document, and it is illicit. If you have companions that you need to impart to, it would be ideal if you respect the designer's diligent work and direct them to buy their own duplicate The Design Space programming does not peruse PDF documents. You should change over the example piece pages to .SVG documents so as to bring them into Design Space. There are various approaches to do this. Despite the fact that bringing in the example pieces in pages or gatherings may appear to be enticing, I don't suggest it. Over the long haul, it will be simpler to work with your records if you spare each example piece as a different document. (This will give you a chance to orchestrate the pieces on the slicing mat to lessen the texture utilized, and will be certainly justified regardless of the additional exertion in advance.)

I use Adobe Illustrator to change over my documents. There are other realistic projects accessible on the web. You need one that will peruse a PDF record, and furthermore spare as a SVG document. When you open the PDF document in another program, spare it as another record with another name, so you don't lose your unique, printable example and directions. I name it something like "Popsicle Top 18 Cricut Maker" to differentiate it from my printable documents. (There is additionally a site called PICSVG that I use to make SVG documents from jpg and png records. It's an extraordinary asset to give a shot too.

You just need the diagrams of the example pieces and each piece ought to be spared as an individual SVG record. Utilize the "utilization artboard" check box to keep the measuring right. If an example piece should be cut on a crease, you have to copy that piece, and after that flip it, and join the lines to make one piece. You need to ensure the lines are covered only a hair! Line the two up precisely, so you have the full piece (the Maker will cut a solitary layer of texture there are no folds.) Delete the covering lines and weld the sort out into one shape. Contingent upon how the example piece is arranged on the page, you may need to change or turn a piece or two to get it precisely right. Guarantee each example piece is arranged here and there as per the grain line and you additionally need to ensure they are that way when you cut them.

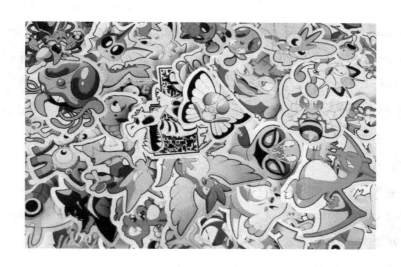

Open Cricut Design Space and make another task. From the left menu, click UPLOAD. Discover your svg records you made on your PC, and transfer them every individually. When they are altogether stacked, add them to your canvas. They will import in dark. I change the shade of the pieces to enable me to keep them all straight. I utilize a different shading for each size doll, and afterward,, guarantee that the pieces that would be cut from different textures are additionally spared in different hues so they will cut on different mats. (For instance, an example that has a top and jeans would have two hues.) Once you have imported your SVGs, set aside the effort to stack a bit of duplicate paper in your cricut machine. Cut out the pieces and contrast them with your printed PDF duplicate to guarantee they are actually the equivalent.

Copy any pieces you have to cut more than one of. One of those should be reflected if they are not the equivalent. For instance, sleeves generally simply should be copied. A bodice back, be that as it may, should be copied with one reflected, so you have a privilege and left back bodice. Rather than bringing in a belt or lash, I just make a square shape in Design Space, giving it a different shading if important to keep it on a different tangle. Some shorts with a front and a back that are different example pieceswill have four different example pieces in your Design Space record. Spare your record so you can utilize it again later!

IT'S EASY TO CUT FABRIC ON THE CRICUT MAKER TO MAKE DOLL CLOTHES.

Lay your texture on your tangle. I like to utilize this device to smooth it out. There are two different ways you can preserve your texture when cutting doll garments on the Cricut Maker. When you hit MAKE IT, you can without much of a stretch move the pieces around and between the mats, yet make certain to keep the pieces arranged accurately for the grain and for directional prints. You can likewise mastermind the pieces before you hit MAKE IT, on your canvas, then ATTACH them to keep their dividing. If you are utilizing the cricut application, attempt the snap tangle where you can put your example pieces straightforwardly on to your formed or pre-cut pieces!

Cut out your example pieces, and sew your doll garments together as indicated by the guidelines. The biggest cricut tangle is 12×24 inches. You may require more than one tangle to cut the majority of your pieces, and most 18 inch doll skirts won't fit on the tangle by any stretch of the imagination. I typically cut the skirt out while the Maker is taking a shot at different pieces and complete both on the double! Here are two cricut packs that will make your tasks somewhat simpler: Cricut Sewing Kit and the Cricut Brayer and Mat Remover Set.

Top Questions Every Cricut Beginner Wants to Know

It is safe to say that you are attempting to choose if you need to purchase a Cricut or are a Cricut learner and confounded on where to begin? You're in the correct spot because prepare to be blown away. The vast majority (myself included) had precisely the same inquiries when beginning. In this way, don't get disappointed and how about we handle the Cricut Beginner FAQ now:

It sounds straightforward, yet I ensure that you will be astonished at the quantity of ventures you can make in a small amount of the time you would almost certainly do them by hand. I'm talking sewing designs, organizer stickers, wooden signs for your home, monogrammed mugs thus considerably more!

This machine is ideal for the imaginative individual who consistently needs to do DIY extends however is lacking in time,, so they sit on your Pinterest load up rather. Also if you have a hand crafted business or Etsy shop, I can practically promise you will get a huge amount of incentive out of this machine.

2. Would i be able to transfer my very own pictures to use with Cricut?

Indeed! You can transfer your very own pictures or any of our free SVG and Me cut records that are now arranged to be absolutely good with Cricut Design Space.

There are a wide range of picture document types out there. The best kind (that we give) are SVGs, which stands (lemme put on my geeky glasses here) versatile vector realistic. Fundamentally, it utilizes math equations to make the picture dependent on focuses between lines. Try not to stress I can see your eyes staring off into the great unknown and won't go in more profundity than that.

The advantage of this is the SVG designs can be broadened without getting that hazy pixelated look you see with other document types, making them totally wonderful for making undertakings of any size!

If you haven't as of now ensure you look at our Free SVG Library which has huge amounts of designs that you can transfer to Design Space today to get making in minutes.

3. What different materials would i be able to cut with Cricut?

Everybody will, in general, consider Cricut machines as cutting paper or vinyl, yet the fact of the matter is there are a LOT more things that a Cricut can cut. Truth be told, the Cricut Explore Air 2 can cut more than 60 sorts of materials!

For example, it can cut chipboard, balsa (very flimsy) wood, magnet material, aluminum (otherwise known as soft drink jars), thus considerably more! For thicker materials, you will need to move up to the profound cut cutting edge for the best cut quality.

Also, the new Cricut Maker can cut EVEN more materials (100+ actually) with 100x the weight intensity of the Explore Air 2. It's strength you inquire? Texture! It has a fresh out of the box new revolving sharp edge which makes it an unquestionable requirement for sewers that can now prepare an undertaking in minutes rather than hours.

Need to see a full rundown of materials and the cutting settings for each? Look at this.

4. What sorts of DIY ventures would i be able to make with a Cricut?

Truly, maybe the best AND most overpowering piece of purchasing a Cricut is that it is SO flexible that you don't have the foggiest idea where to start. In this way, oppose the data over-burden and attempt to concentrate on one anticipate at once.

The amusing thing about Cricut ventures is that, when I was beginning, I will think about a zillion undertakings or see some on Pinterest and think "hello, I wanna make that!" Then, I plunk down to make a task, and my brain would go absolutely clear!

Indeed, to help with this, I thought of a HUGE rundown of Cricut ventures (that will keep on developing so continue returning for updates). You can peruse through, pick one from the rundown, and get creating in a matter of moments! Also, it presently accompanies a FREE printable adaptation you can allude to for motivation. Along these lines, ensure you head over and download that if you don't have it.

5. Will it be simple for me to figure out how to utilize Cricut Design Space to make my very own custom activities?

That's right, and I'm here to help! Look at our Cricut instructional exercises page here, which is a great spot for amateurs to begin! We include new recordings every week and even give accommodating free assets and agendas so ensure you return frequently.

You don't have to claim a Cricut to begin rehearsing with Design Space. When you get your machine, you'll be a stage ahead!

6. What supplies do I have to begin?

This is one of the inquiries I had the hardest time replying as a fledgling. I scanned for a printable asset on the web and was stunned when I couldn't discover one – so I chose to make my own to impart to you!

I took a huge amount of time inquiring about, getting counsel from others, and afterward accumulating this tremendous rundown of Essential Cricut Supplies Every Beginner Should Have that I am offering to you (fortunate duck) to spare all of you the time it took me

It will ceaselessly be refreshed, so ensure you inquire intermittently to ensure you have the most recent rendition. Likewise, let me know if you have any sacred goal Cricut items or tips that I ought to incorporate!

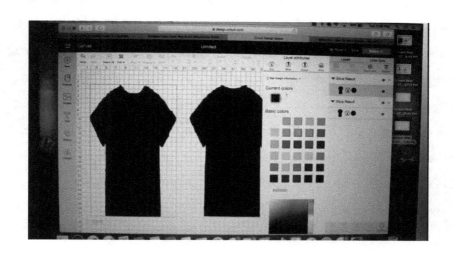

73

IS BUYING A CRICUT WORTH IT?

I was visiting with a companion a day or two ago who was thinking about purchasing a Cricut Explore. At $299 ($249 at a bargain!), it is anything but an economical buy and she was thinking about whether she'd use it enough to justify the cost. I believe it's a substantial inquiry if you're pondering purchasing a Cricut. So I needed to discuss the reasons that it's an incredible buy — and several reasons you should need to pause.

MOTIVATIONS TO BUY A CRICUT

I've said this a couple of times in different posts, yet when I initially found out about the Cricut I truly thought I had no utilization for such a machine. I thought it was primarily for scrapbookers and since I didn't scrapbook, I never investigated. In any case, seeing it in real life live, getting a Cricut myself, and working with the Cricut group throughout the most recent three years, I've come to understand this is completely probably the best apparatus I claim for making a wide range of things. These are a couple of my preferred motivations to purchase a Cricut, however there are numerous a lot additionally relying upon your needs!

To begin with, the Cricut Explore is so unimaginably flexible. I realize I make a ton of undertakings here that are specifically for the blog and designed to rouse you to make things all alone. Be that as it may, I am additionally always utilizing it for ventures that never come around here. Just as of late I've made marks for provisions in my art room, craftsmanship for the kid's room, confetti, custom tote sacks and diaries for our ladies' retreat, shirts for a companion's child's first birthday celebration party, improvements for a Bunco party, vinyl names for an infant shower support, shirts for a Firefly-themed party, and a few other arbitrary cut documents for companions. I cherish that I can make such a large number of sorts of tasks with the Cricut and that I can utilize my Cricut and cunning abilities to assist my less-shrewd companions with their activities.

Second, it will spare you so much time. If you're utilized to hand cutting, the Cricut can do it so a lot quicker and better — and it will spare your hands (my hands spasm so gravely with scissors!). I can't accept the amount more I can do because my Cricut makes making quicker. Our gatherings have a great time components because I can make things quite a lot more rapidly than designing and cutting by hand. Furthermore, I get the opportunity to do ventures that I never would have managed without the Cricut, such as making custom names for the majority of my flavor containers — it is extremely unlikely I'd at any point cut those mind boggling letters by hand!

Third, you can make your very own custom tasks. My preferred component of the Cricut Explore is having the option to transfer my very own designs. Nearly all that I make is customized precisely how I need it and it makes all that I make feel considerably more uncommon. You can likewise utilize it to customize gifts — getting a birthday present is extraordinary, yet getting one tweaked with your name is far superior!

Also, fourth, it's not difficult to learn. I figure individuals can be a little overpowered with a machine that accompanies a product they've never utilized. In any case, the Cricut Design Space is easy to use and there are a huge amount of Make It Now extends that have a little expectation to absorb information. Indeed, there are further developed things you can do with the Cricut that will set aside some effort to adapt, yet there are instructional exercises everywhere throughout the Internet on the most proficient method to utilize the machine and the product (counting here on my blog!), and Cricut backing is useful too. If you're terrified of the expectation to absorb information, don't be — simply set aside some effort to become acquainted with the machine and the product, make a couple of basic ventures, and watch YouTube instructional exercises if you're trapped. Try not to give learning the machine a chance to stop you from getting one!

In any case, we should be genuine. In fact practically any undertaking you can do with a Cricut you could without one. Be that as it may, the Cricut will do it So. Much. Better. Your undertakings will look progressively proficient, you'll spare yourself a thousand cerebral pains, you won't squander as much material, and it will be a gobzillion times quicker. I've been making as long as I can remember and this is the primary apparatus that has, and this isn't exaggeration, altered the manner in which I create. It spares personal time, stress, and cash and those things merit everything to me nowadays. I think the Cricut is absolutely justified, despite all the trouble to nearly any individual who wants to create, just as individuals like educators (who need to remove 30 whatevers for their understudies), mothers (who need to customize things for their littles), and even specialists (like model plane developers who need many-sided decals).

REASONS NOT TO BUY A CRICUT

As much as I truly accept that the Cricut is a magnificent making apparatus that you can utilize constantly, I thought of a couple of situations where you should need to hold off getting one. I'm a major adherent to just purchasing what you're going to utilize, and it benefits nobody in any way to have a machine that they never really create with!

In the first place, you must have some craving to be a creator. You could love all the charming things on the planet, however if it's only simpler for you to get it on Etsy because you don't have a craving for making it yourself, your Cricut will sit unused. I do accept that the Cricut makes making and making a whoooole parcel simpler and you don't should be excessively inventive to utilize it since Cricut Access and the Make It Now tasks give you access to such a significant number of extraordinary thoughts. In any case, if you would prefer not to make stuff, you're not really going to make stuff. Am I right?

The second reason you might not have any desire to purchase a Cricut is if you're one of those individuals who simply purchase things because they are cool (indeed, a Cricut is VERY cool). You know your identity! I used to be one of these individuals. I had boxes of cool items, instruments, and supplies that I never utilized. Things sat in boxes and accumulated residue until one day I chose to cleanse everything out of my specialty room that I didn't effectively utilize. It felt so great however I likewise felt regretful for having so much abundance. Be straightforward with yourself. Regardless of whether you adore the possibility of a Cricut, would you say you are really going to remove it from the container and use it? Is it going to be a piece of your ordinary making day? If in this way, get one. If not, don't squander your cash. A Cricut does nothing simply sitting in a case social occasion dust.

Third is if you extremely simply love cutting stuff by hand. I may believe you're insane and it makes my hands throb simply pondering it — however if that is your thing, put it all on the line!

These reasons are alright! I'd preferably you not feel remorseful for owning a machine that you never use. I'd preferably you spend your cash on something that you will utilize and that will bring you bliss.

Things you Need to Know before Buying one

The Cricut is an extraordinary machine for individuals that affection making, and for or individuals that need to cut a great deal of things and different kinds of materials.

Before I got my Cricut I had TONS and TONS of inquiries. Truth be told! Despite everything I do. That is the reason I am making this monster post so I can archive and spare you the a long stretch of time of research I have done.

In the wake of perusing this incredibly and complete guide you will know if a Cricut Machine is an ideal choice for you!

Is it accurate to say that you are prepared?

This is arrangement of inquiries I had when I purchased my Cricut. I truly wish I approached this kind of substance you are going to peruse. It would've made my life so a lot simpler!

After you are finished perusing this post. You will know without a doubt whether the Cricut is the correct decision for you or not.

These inquiries go from easy to progressively difficult. Subsequently you will gain proficiency with about this machine as you go!

A few inquiries are much increasingly broad and they really require an additional post for it. So if there's a connection to one specific inquiry and you need to get familiar with that subject, simply snap to find out additional.

1. Do I truly require a Cricut?

A Cricut is a cutting machine and is a blessing from heaven for some, crafters out there. You can utilize it for various different things like card making, home stylistic layout, and so forth.

Do you art or wind up in a position where you have to cut a ton? If the response to that is yes. Then you will absolutely profit by having a Cricut. Be that as it may, if you are not into cunning things. Let's be honest! a Cricut isn't something you will truly profit by.

2. Are there different machines that can do something very similar?

Indeed! There are numerous different alternatives you can discover there that can do what the Cricut does to some broaden.

In the market there are two other real brands that likewise cut an extraordinary assortment of materials and that additionally have incredible audits.

These brands are: Silhouette America and Brother.

3. Is the Cricut superior to anything different machines out there?

I accept each bite the dust cutting machine is astounding.

How would I realize that?

It's straightforward. If you take a gander at all of their audits on Amazon you will see that essentially every one of them have multiple begins.

That says that regardless of what machine you pick you will totally adore it

Here's the other thing. Because I happen to have a Cricut and I adore it, I am not going to diss on different brands or machines.

Cricut happens to be the pass on slicing machine brand I chose to go to with. So essentially all you see here will be towards this specific brand

4. For what reason Should I pick Cricut over different brands?

Because it's the one you need.

A few people will say they abhor it, other individuals will say they cherish it. Yet, toward the day's end the cash is leaving your pocket. So you ought to pick what you are progressively OK with.

I for one imagine that Provo Craft and Novelty – the organization that made this stunning instrument – is a slick organization and you can see and feel the nature of their items. You realize that all that they make is made with affection.

Their machines improve inevitably; however they likewise think of new devices and embellishments that make things so a lot simpler and pleasant. You can genuinely grow your breaking points and innovativeness with these machines.

One of different things I have loved about this machine, and that I really discovered after I got it is that the Cricut is in excess of a shaper!

There's the Cricut Community. You can get huge amounts of thoughts and free instructional exercises on the web. We creatives love sharing tips and traps on the best way to exploit this very cool apparatus.

5. For what reason did I get a Cricut?

Not that this inquiry matters to you. In any case, this is the fundamental reason I got one, and you may feel roused by it!

I recall a discussion with my relative where I was asking her what should I blog about. She realizes I make and design beautiful things for basically any event.

In the wake of giving me huge amounts of thoughts; She prescribed me to find out about the Cricut!

The seed was planted. I read huge amounts of instructional exercises, surveys! What's more, a few months after the fact. I GOT ONE!

So for me it was my relative sentiment. She has companions that adoration the machine. So if you know somebody that as of now utilizes a kick the bucket cutting machine and they adore it. Simply take their statement.

Furthermore, if you don't know anybody…

All things considered, Trust me when I state that the Cricut Machine is the best thing out there. You won't be frustrated!

. What are the accessible Cricut Machines out there?

I am going to separate this for you extremely simple! At this moment you there are 3 different models of Cricut Machines accessible:

Cricut Explore Family: These are the most widely recognized machines and they have 3 different alternatives for you to browse. These three machines can cut similar materials, But every one of them have different highlights.

Cricut Explore One: First conceived of the Explore family and just has one apparatus holder so you cut and draw independently.

Cricut Explore Air: Has Bluetooth (This is an absolute necessity for me I don't care for having a string append to my PC) and both device holders so you can cut and draw simultaneously!

Cricut Explore Air 2: Has similar capacities, that the investigate air however it's multiple times quicker.

Cricut Maker: This machine is their most recent discharge and you can cut thick materials like calfskin and even a few kinds of wood.

Cricut Cuttlebug: this is the main Cricut that can formally embellish. Remember that this machine doesn't approach the Cricut Design Space, or any web at all. It's an essential however incredible shaper.

There were different machines accessible also. Furthermore, you may almost certainly buy them on amazon or utilized. Notwithstanding, they are not good with Cricut Design Space and the product they utilized before – Cricut Craft Room – has been closed down totally.

So simply don't purchase any of the old forms. It resembles purchasing a spic and span I-telephone 4. OK do that?

All through this post, except if I notice the Cricut Cuttlebug, most inquiries will be responded in due order regarding the Cricut Explore Family and Cricut Maker.

7. Is the Cricut excessively costly?

Ideal off bat let me reveal to you that YES a Cricut machine can be very costly.

In any case, see I state that it very well may be. This is because if you take a gander at a portion of the primary machines you can see that there are great arrangements and you can begin when you need.

The most affordable machine is the Cricut Cuttlebug – A little however incredible machine – and the Most costly choice is for their most recent discharge, The Cricut Maker.

Look at costs and correlation for the Cricut Explore Family and Cricut Maker

8. Is the Cricut justified, despite all the trouble?

This is so factor and it needs to do about your diversions, needs and furthermore your financial limit.

If you make once per year, listen to me you DON'T require a Cricut. Notwithstanding, if making and making stuff is your jam then a Cricut merits each penny.

You additionally need to see life through your need focal points. For what reason do I say this. Because life is about priorities.\; each choice we make in life ought to be lined up with that.

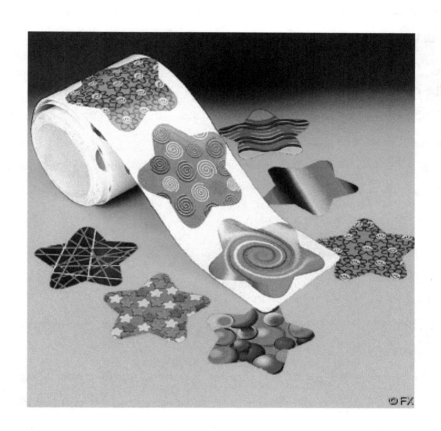

Is having a Cricut going to profit you and make your life simple enough to spare time – time is cash – and simply make your life progressively charming?

If your answer is YES: Then GO pull the trigger.

I am not the sort of individual that purchases everything. Be that as it may, now and again when I weight upsides and downsides. I simply put it all on the line.

9. What is the best Cricut I can get?

The best Cricut you can get. Pass on is the Cricut Maker.

It's their most up to date discharge and they are concocting numerous devices that will make cutting and making very simple and way progressively pleasant. As it were the Cricut Maker is a definitive Crafter's fantasy.

10. What is the best Cricut for me?

The best Cricut you can get is the one that meets these 3 things:

The one you can bear.

The one you can slice the materials you need to cut.

The one that will leave you with extra cash to purchase materials (regularly overlooked).

This is the reason I got the Air Explore 2 rather than the Cricut Maker.

Most importantly I couldn't bear the cost of the creator. Second of all – as of now in life – I am just keen on cutting paper, vinyl and some texture to a great extent. Furthermore, to wrap things up, what is the purpose of having an increasingly costly machine if you don't have the cash to purchase additional materials to work with?

In any case, if you haven't purchased a machine and you truly need to cut wood and texture I believe is smarter to do the speculation now, and after that get additional apparatuses and materials as you go.

Update: Eventually, I got the Cricut Maker also because I needed to show all of you the conceivable outcomes with the two machines.

11. Would it be a good idea for me to overhaul my Cricut?

If you as of now have a Cricut machine given me a chance to reveal to you something – You ROCK!

Is it true that you are thinking about in updating? I feel you after I purchased my Explore Air 2 I felt deficient, every one of the instructional exercises are currently for the Maker, and that I should simply overhaul.

Isn't that SO SILLY?

Do you redesign your telephone, vehicle, and other electronic gadgets consistently? I sure don't. So – except if I am given one – until I misuse each and every plausibility and I am prepared to learn different strategies. I won't overhaul my machine.

Shouldn't something be said about you?

Would you like to overhaul because you need the most up to date form? Or then again, would you like to update because you really exceeded your present machine?

If you said yes to the second and have the spending limit for it! Welcome to the Cricut Maker family! I am in no uncertainty that you will observe this machine to be an incredible fit for you

12. Where Can I get the Cricut?

There are MANY spots where you can get this machine.

You can think that its essentially at any specialty store like Michael's and JOANN. Indeed, even some Walmart Stores have it accessible. So if you need to begin today you can drive and get it there.

I for one cherish shopping on Cricut's site because that is the place I locate the best arrangements.

13. Does the Cricut and Cricut Materials ever go on Sale?

That's right!

Cricut has things on Sale practically constantly.

You can discover great ones during the occasions and exceptional events. A few retailers additionally run incredible limits. Truth be told I see huge amounts of them on Facebook.

14. Where would i be able to locate the best deals and arrangements for the Cricut?

If I were going to buy a Cricut right now I would do it from their Official Website. They simply have extraordinary limits accessible constantly.

Here you can discover incredible arrangements on packs, machines, and materials.

15. What materials would i be able to cut with the Cricut?

There are hundreds – actually – of materials you can cut with these astonishing machine these are some of them:

Plan Paper

A wide range of cardstock

Metallic Paper

Vinyl (Iron on, sparkle, lasting, removable)

Texture and materials

Artificial Leather

Ridged Paper

Meager Woods (Cricut Maker as it were)

Sticker Paper

Material Paper

And the sky is the limit from there!

16. Where would i be able to get Cricut materials?

You can get materials in your preferred Craft Store. Much the same as you would get the Cricut.

I am truly astonished at all of the alternatives you can discover on the web. Amazon has hundreds if not a great many choices for you to buy.

The Cricut site likewise has cool materials, yet they just offer their very own image. Be that as it may, my preferred spot to get materials is Michaels; I adore strolling through the isles, I can truly invests huge amounts of energy (and cash ahhg) there.

17. Are Cricut materials costly?

Contingent upon the undertakings you need to cut, Cricut Materials can be very costly. This is the reason you should buy the machine that will likewise enable you to purchase things to cut.

It's silly for you to get the Cricut Maker if you wont have an additional spending limit for you to cut different materials. That resembles purchasing Snow Tires when you live in Florida, and there's no Snow. Get my point?

Easily overlooked details to a great extent, truly include. Materials like basswood can be over the top expensive too.

At the present time, I am concentrating more on paper, and I will move my way up. Paper is the most ideal route for you to gain proficiency with your machine because if you cut something incorrectly is simply paper. So it is anything but a major ordeal if you mess it up.

18. Would i be able to use off brand materials to use with my Cricut?

Truly, indeed, yes!

You don't need to be constrained to the materials that Cricut makes. There are hundreds if not a large number of astonishing materials you can get on the web or on your preferred Craft store.

I am certain that with time there will be considerably more alternatives.

19. What is the Cricut riddle box and how can it work?

Consistently Cricut discharges a Mystery Box!

This container is load up with astonishing materials yet you truly don't have the foggiest idea what they are. It's an amazement till you get that crate!

The astounding thing about this crate is that you will get more than what you really paid. What I mean by this is if you were going to purchase the majority of the materials that come in the crate independently the cost would be so a lot higher.

They do run out. So try to get yours toward the start of every month!

20. What is the Cricut versatile device System?

The Cricut Adaptive System is an amazingly and ground-breaking highlight that lone the Cricut Maker has. This element controls the heading and of the edge at untouched. Actually, This apparatus is stunning to the point that it can modify the weight of the cutting edge to coordinate the materials you are working with!

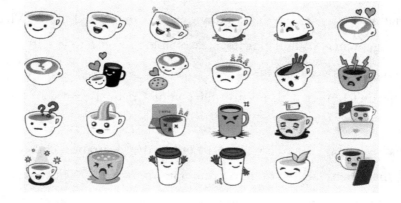

This innovation is the thing that enables the Cricut Maker to cut with 10X more power than any of the other Cricut Explore Family machines. This is the reason the Maker can cut thick materials like wood and cowhide.

Cool. Isn't that so?

21. Does the Cricut print?

The Cricut Machine doesn't print. Be that as it may, the majority of the present machines they offer – Except Cuttlebug – have a choice to draw and diagram things like letters, shapes, and so on.

If you as of now have a Cricut, this inquiry appears to be so self-evident. Be that as it may, I had this inquiry before I purchased mine. What's more, I genuinely couldn't locate a reasonable response to it.

22. Does the Cricut need ink?

You needn't bother with ink to utilize your Cricut. Because it doesn't print.

Be that as it may, if you are going to utilize the illustration choice. you need their pens so as to have the option to draw. They have an extraordinary assortment of alternatives for you to look over.

23. Does the Cricut Laminate?

No. The Cricut Machines don't overlay. Wouldn't it be decent, however?

24. Does the Cricut Emboss?

The main Cricut Machine that can really decorate is the Cricut Cuttlebug. This is the thing that the official site says: "The main Cricut® machine that can embellish, the Cricut Cuttlebug™gives proficient looking outcomes with spotless, fresh cuts and profound, even decorates."

Be that as it may, you can discover workarounds and make stencils with any of different machines and decorate essentially anything your heart wants. While I was examining this inquiry, I discovered huge amounts of cool instructional exercises on YouTube that show you how to do it! This was my top choice.

25. Does the Cricut Sew?

No. The Cricut doesn't sew. It's so natural to feel that it does because you hear the majority of the beneficial things that you can do if you are a sewer.

26. Does the Cricut cut texture?

Truly, the Cricut can cut texture.

If you work with textures and need to cut huge amounts of texture in different sizes, the Cricut will be your best and increasingly confided in Cutting partner.

The Cricut producer enables you to cut texture with no fortified material. Along these lines, if sewing is your calling and this is the principle explanation behind you to get a Cricut. I will very prescribe to put resources into the Maker.

You can cut Fabric with the Any of the Cricut Explore Family machines. Notwithstanding, the texture should be reinforced. I will clarify better in the following inquiry.

27. What on the planet is a support material, and how can it identify with cutting texture?

Would you be able to trust I couldn't locate an average response to this? Fortunately, I am here to clarify you what this implies

The Cricut Explore Family machines and the Cricut Maker can cut texture. Be that as it may, there's a major proviso and that will be that with the end goal for you to have the option to cut texture with the Explore Family machines you need a support material.

Support – or otherwise called Heat and Bond – in the Cricut and pass on cutting machines world is a sort of material that enables you to settle textures on the cutting mat. As such, If you don't hold fast this material to your textures when utilizing the Cricut Explore Machines, your textures won't get cut up appropriately, and they will get destroyed and additionally extended.

Dreadful right?

28. Does the Cricut cut wood?

Truly and No. Out of all the cutting machines that Cricut has accessible. Just the Cricut Maker can cut wood. A portion of the kinds of wood you can cut are balsa and basswood.

You likewise need to remember that the Cricut Maker itself with the typical cutting edge that accompanies DOES NOT cut wood. For these sort of task, you will require the Knife Blade, which is a sort cutting edge that is specifically designed to cut thick materials.

29. What are a portion of the undertakings I can do with a Cricut Machine?

There are numerous activities you can make with a Cricut machine! This is only a modest rundown of a portion of the things you can achieve. Note: Links on this area are a portion of my Cricut instructional exercises.

Home Decoration: Decals for your windows, dividers. Or on the other hand, something that I like a great deal is to customize things like crates, or even your cooking flavors.

Stickers: for arranging, journaling, and that's only the tip of the iceberg

Welcome Cards: You can make top of the line welcome cards. Like those, you find in the store!

Garments Items: Cut and iron on beautiful and customized designs on your T-Shirts.

3D Projects: like gift boxes and even paper toys! –

With the Cricut Maker, you can cut wood and make 3D and tough ventures.

Cut texture and make design things for your dress and the sky is the limit from there.

Your creative mind is the utmost!

30. What on the planet are Cricut cartridges and Do I need them?

The word cartridge in the Cricut world is different than in the printing scene; I feel that is the reason I figured the Cricut could print!

Fundamentally Cricut Cartridges are a lot of pictures, designs or textual styles you can buy and get the chance to keep until the end of time. They are normally designed around a specific subject, for example, Disney, Pop Corn gathering, and anything you can essentially consider.

There are 2 kinds of cartridges. Physical and Digital, the physical ones can be embedded in the machine. Also, the Digital ones you can legitimately buy from the Cricut site or Cricut Design Space.

When you initiate the cartridges, they will be accessible to you on the product, and the physical variants are never again required.

I get the inclination that the Physical Cartridges will be ceased sooner or later. A major confirmation of this is the Cricut Maker – their most recent discharge – doesn't have a space for you to embed them. (You have to purchase a connector for this)

31. What is Cricut Infusible Ink?

Cricut Infusible Ink is a sort of innovation that permits to you make and move your designs to a base material. What makes this innovation so interesting is that the Infusible Ink move will end up one with the base material you pick.

The outcomes in the wake of applying Cricut Infusible ink are stunning and amazingly high caliber. They are consistently smooth, don't ring endlessly, and they will remain in your base material until the end of time.

32. What on the planet are Cricut Mats and which one do I need?

You have no clue the majority of the migraines I got attempting to make sense of this!

A Cricut Mat is the surface you use with the goal for you to have the option to cut specific materials. They come in 2 different sizes: 12 x 12 and 12 x 24 inches.

The Cricut Mats are sticky and depending of the material you are going to cut you are in an ideal situation utilizing different degrees of stickiness. Or then again otherwise called a holds.

As of now there are 4 sorts of mats:

Light Grip (Blue)

Solid Grip (Purple)

Standard Grip (Green)

Texture Grip (Pink)

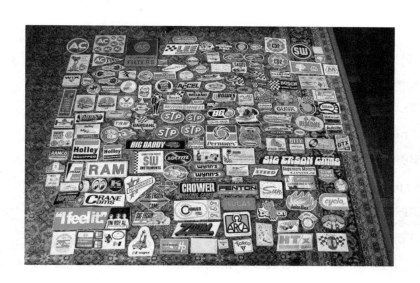

When I initially got my Cricut, I got a pleasant pack on Amazon that incorporated the 4 mats.

If you are simply beginning. The best MAT for you is the standard grasp. The more grounded the hold, the heavier the material you can utilize.

For example it you are cutting ordinary and dainty paper you would utilize a Light Grip tangle, however, if you are anticipating cutting a heavier material like thick Cardstock you are in an ideal situation with a Strong Grip tangle.

Essentially every machine accompanies a Standard Grip Mat. Ensure you read the portrayal of the items before you purchase.

If you need to adapt more top to bottom about Cricut Mats make a point to peruse this book. It will indicate you all that you have to know.

33. What is a Cricut Blade and which one do I need?

The cutting edge is the thing that cuts the materials. lol Right?

Be that as it may, there's something significant for you to know, before you begin and if you are anticipating cutting thicker materials

Right now there are 5 cutting edges accessible. Every sharp edge has different capacities and is fit to cut different materials.

Fine Point Blade: Ideal for light and medium materials like paper, vinyl and cardstock. It comes now in a gold shading.

Profound Point Blade: Great for thick materials like chipboard, thick cardstock, froth sheets, and so forth.

Fortified Fabric Blade: Ideal for cutting texture! Texture should be fortified with support material.

Revolving Blade (Only for the Cricut Maker): Cuts practically any kind of texture and the texture can be simply place on the tangle. It accompanies the Maker and at the minutes it's not sold separately. Be that as it may, they do sell the revolving substitution unit

Knife Blade (Only for the Cricut Maker): This great little edge can cut exceptionally thick materials like basswood!

So if wood is your jam, then the Cricut Maker + the Knife cutting edge are an unquestionable requirement.

If you need to become familiar with the majority of the Cricut Blades and their differences, read this extreme guide

34. What edges accompany each Cricut Machine?

When you purchase only a machine (No pack) the generally accompany a cutting edge. How about we see what cutting edge accompanies each machine!

Cricut Explore One: fine point cutting edge

Cricut Explore Air: fine point edge

Cricut Explore Air 2: fine point sharp edge

Cricut Maker: Rotary sharp edge, fine point cutting edge

35. To what extent does the Cricut Blade Last?

Cricut Blades keep going relying upon the material and recurrence you use them.

There's not by any stretch of the imagination a specific time for it. If you see your materials aren't being cut with a similar freshness and facilitate that they used to. Then it's the ideal opportunity for you to supplant it.

36. What Other Cricut Accessories do I need?

This is a dubious inquiry, and It thoroughly relies upon the sort of materials you need to work with and cut.

Despite the fact that the Cricut machines are equipped for some things, you have to utilize it with the correct apparatuses to genuinely make it work. For example, if you have any of the Explore Family Machines and need to cut texture, you have to ensure that you have:

Sponsorship Material

Texture Bonded – Blade

Standard Grip Mat

Then again if you need to cut texture with the creator you can likewise utilize the above apparatus, or you can pick a rotating sharp edge in addition to a Fabric Grip Mat.

Most normal and light weight materials can be cut with the Fine Point Blade (The cutting edge that accompanies each machine) and the Standard grasp Mat.

Be that as it may, as you investigate and become increasingly mindful of your machine and the materials you are utilizing, things will turn out to be a great deal more simpler!

I know it's precarious however once you get the hang of it you will be a specialist. The beneficial thing about this machine is that when you are going to cut a specific material, the program will let you know precisely what materials you need!

Cool right?

Another significant thing here and something that I consider critical is to get is a portion of the their extraordinary devices.

There are various sets for you to look over. Be that as it may, the most well-known are the Basic, and the Essential Tool set.

37. Is it better for me to get a pack or simply the machine?

If you visit the Cricut Online Store, Amazon, and other online retailers you will see that there huge amounts of packs you can buy.

I really got a group myself from Amazon. They are great worth and accompanied a beginning pack for you to begin as quickly as time permits.

When you are searching for packs, ensure they incorporate what you need to begin with.

For example, if you are simply going to begin cutting vinyl and paper. The ideal pack for you will incorporate your preferred machine + some vinyl sheets + standard grasp tangle + essential toolbox. (This is the thing that I got)

Nonetheless, if your fundamental intention is to cut texture. You need a pack that accompanies the fundamentals for you to begin. Like sewing instruments and so on.

If you get the Cricut Maker they have extraordinary choices for you to begin cutting texture.

38. Is there something different I need other than the Cricut and Accessories:

There are different things you need and there are regularly not referenced:

Materials you need to cut and learn with. I will prescribe you to rehearse with paper tons and tons before you choose to cut something like texture or wood that can be increasingly costly.

Persistence: It's an expectation to learn and adapt... Not all things will come simple, however will turn out to be simple

YouTube gorge instructional exercises for you to totally ace this machine – I am anticipating putting TONS of stunning instructional exercises. If you like this post make a point to buy in (It's likewise an incredible manner to help my work)

39. What on the planet is a Cricut Easy Press?

A Cricut Easy Press is a cool gadget that permits you move your Iron On vinyl to T-shirts, sweaters, blankets and that's just the beginning! It comes in 3 different sizes and you can get the one that addresses your issues:

The sizes are:

9×9 Inches: This size is incredible to move designs to Adult size T-Shirts

6×7 Inches: Ideal to press on little bits of dress like onesies and other infant garments.

10×12 Inches: Perfect to Iron on in enormous surfaces like blankets and covers.

40. Is the Cricut Easy Press extremely justified, despite all the trouble?

This is a Yes and No answer, for me the appropriate response tilts more to the no extremely justified, despite all the trouble.

The principle reason is because I can simply utilize my customary iron; and since I am not completing a great deal of iron on activities right now It doesn't generally bode well for me to contribute on it.

41. Is the Cricut simple to utilize?

Everything in life has an expectation to learn and adapt.

When my Cricut arrived I felt a smidgen overpowered I admit! It very well may threaten from the start, yet once you get its hang. I am certain those staggering days will be only relics of days gone by.

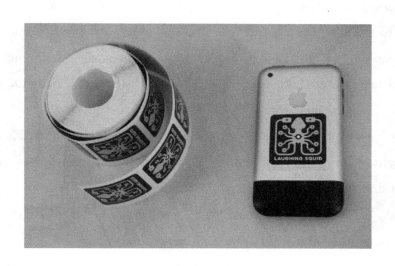

So the principle believe is to stay with it. Watch the same number of YouTube channels (I am making my own) and Instagram recordings you can. Search for instructional exercises! I will put EVERYTHING you have to know. No doubt

Try not to overwhelm.... . We are in the data age, and information is earnestly at the tip of a google search.

42. Do I should be a technically knowledgeable to have the option to utilize the Cricut?

You don't should be super, technically knowledgeable. Anyway, you do need to know a few nuts and bolts and fundamentals about the manner in which the PCs work. For example, you have to realize how to function PCs a tad. Things Like opening a page and login into Cricut Design Space – Where you organize the thing you have to cut.

If you have a Smart telephone and need to work your machine inside the application. You likewise should be natural on the most proficient method to download the application.

Do you believe you won't most likely learn it? Try not to feel like that! The sky is the limit if you put the time and exertion.

I am here perking you up. Additionally, I have the majority of the aim of making this learning open to you!

43. What is the Cricut perfect with?

All together for your machine to work, you should be associated with the Cricut Design Space.

The Cricut Design Space is just perfect with Windows and Mac working frameworks. At the end of the day; you need a personal computer with the end goal for you to utilize the Cricut Machines.

If you need to utilize your machine without web, you have to download the Cricut Design Space application. This application is very helpful, and it interface by means of Bluetooth.

This application is accessible just for iOS a.k.a Iphone and Apple clients. In any case, if you are an Android client, don't lose trust! Cricut just discharged a beta alternative and in spite of the fact that It doesn't have every one of the abilities you would have on an Iphone. I am almost certain one day it will arrive.

44. Would i be able to associate my Cricut by means of Bluetooth to my telephone or PC?

It relies upon the machine you have.

The Explore Air, Explore Air 2, and Maker have worked in Bluetooth innovation so they can associate with your work area or telephone.

For the Cricut Explore One you will require a connector to have the option to interface your Cricut through Bluetooth to your PC or telephone. If you as of now have this machine I believe is something great to have.

In any case, if you're simply inquiring about what machine is ideal, I would recommend to begin looking from the Explore Air or more.

NOTE: The Cricut Cuttlebug doesn't have any electronic or Bluetooth abilities.

45. Do I need Internet for me to utilize the Cricut?

If you are wanting to utilize your Cricut from your PC, you NEED to have Internet get to. Notwithstanding, the Cricut Design App – Available for iOS and Android telephones – will permit to utilize your Cricut machine disconnected.

46. Is there an elective Software to utilize the Cricut?

Probably not!

Obviously, there was a path for you to do it with an outsider program; however, it's not accessible with the fresher machines.

What I for one do is that I design what I have to Cut on Illustrator, and afterward I cut it on my printer. In any case, if it's simply content and essential shapes. The Cricut Design Space is simply enough.

47. How does the Cricut work?

So far you've found out about the Cricut itself. Things like the mats, cutting edges, materials, and what the machines are perfect with.

However, how does the Cricut really work? For the Cricut Machine to cut, you have to utilize it alongside the Cricut Design Space. This is where you'll lay and sort out your design to be cut.

48. What is Cricut Design Space?

The Cricut Design Space is the product that enables you to compose, make, lastly cut your undertakings. Without the Design Space you can't work your machine. That is for what reason is significant for you to figure out how to utilize it.

The Cricut Machine is extraordinary yet if you don't figure out how to utilize the Design Space, it resembles purchasing a camera and not taking photographs. Or then again purchasing a Smart Phone and not making a telephone or video call.

49. Is Cricut Design Space Free?

Indeed!

All things considered, if you have machine is free

You can transfer your very own designs to be cut. You can even access your framework's textual styles and a few shapes to make straightforward cuts for nothing.

What's not free is Cricut Access.

50. What is Cricut Access?

Cricut Access is a GIANT library that will enable you to choose and make officially designed activities. This is helpful it you are simply beginning.

When you have Cricut Access and relying upon the arrangement you have, you can choose one of a kind text styles, illustrations, 3D Projects, and if you can think it, they have it.

They have ventures for any event and any materials you like to work with. It's very great.

CONCLUSION

The Cricut cutting machine is as astonishing as it is because of Cricut Design Space, the free application that causes the enchantment to occur. And keeping in mind that Cricut Design Space is entirely simple and easy to use, acing it doesn't occur without any forethought.

That is for what reason I'm here to share my most loved Cricut Design Space instructional exercises, tips, and traps with you! These will change your Cricut life!